Table of Contents

1 Introduction to Parasitism

Parasitism, at its core, is a biological relationship where one organism, the parasite, benefits at the expense of another, the host. This interaction isn't simply a matter of one organism consuming another; it's a complex interplay of adaptation, survival, and evolution. Parasites have evolved an astounding array of strategies to exploit their hosts, often resulting in significant harm, even death. Understanding this intricate relationship forms the foundation for tackling parasitic diseases.

The diversity within the parasitic world is breathtaking. From single-celled protozoa like Plasmodium falciparum, the causative agent of malaria, to multicellular helminths such as tapeworms and hookworms, the spectrum is vast. Their size, their life cycles, and the tissues they infect are all incredibly varied. Some parasites are highly specialized, infecting only a single host species, while others have broad host ranges, infecting a variety of animals including humans. This diversity necessitates a nuanced approach to understanding and treating parasitic infections. Each parasite presents a unique challenge.

Understanding how parasites invade human cells is critical. Active penetration involves the parasite actively breaching cellular barriers using mechanical forces or enzymes that degrade host tissues. This process demands significant energy expenditure from the parasite, but it provides direct access to the host's cellular machinery. Conversely, passive entry utilizes pre-existing openings or vulnerabilities in the host's defenses. This method can be significantly more efficient, relying on the host's own processes for entry. More insidious still is cellular hijacking, whereby parasites manipulate cellular processes to their advantage, essentially using the host's own mechanisms to facilitate their own invasion and survival.

The immune system, our body's defense force, is constantly engaged in a battle against invading pathogens. Parasites, however, have evolved cunning strategies to evade this response. Antigenic variation is a remarkable example. Parasites can change the surface proteins they display, effectively becoming invisible to the immune system's memory cells. This constant shifting of identity allows them to continually evade detection and eradication. Immune suppression is another powerful tactic, actively hindering the immune response. Some parasites release molecules that suppress the host's immune cells, creating a permissive environment for their own survival and propagation. This intricate interplay between parasite and host immune system shapes the course of infection.

The clinical manifestations of parasitic infections are incredibly diverse. Symptoms range from mild discomfort to severe organ damage or even death, depending on the parasite and the host's immune response. Malaria, for instance, can manifest as flu-like symptoms or progress to severe cerebral malaria, a life-threatening condition. Similarly, intestinal helminth infections might present with mild abdominal discomfort, while others can cause severe malnutrition and anemia. Accurate diagnosis relies on identifying the specific parasite, which can involve microscopic examination of blood or stool samples, serological tests, or even molecular techniques like PCR. The complexity of disease presentation necessitates a thorough understanding of the disease progression to guide appropriate treatment. Therapeutic strategies vary significantly depending on the parasite involved. Antimalarial drugs, such as artemisinin-based combination therapies (ACTs), are highly effective against Plasmodium species. However, drug resistance is a major concern, constantly driving the need for new drug development. Beyond malaria, a wide array of antiparasitic drugs target various other parasites. These drugs interfere with metabolic processes crucial for parasite survival or directly attack the parasite's structural components. However, similar challenges with drug resistance apply, making the development and implementation of new treatments an ongoing necessity. The selection pressure exerted by these drugs invariably leads to the evolution of resistant parasite strains.

The relationship between parasites and their hosts is a constant evolutionary arms race. Parasites constantly adapt and evolve to overcome host defenses, while hosts, in turn, develop stronger immune responses. This coevolutionary process has shaped both parasite and host biology in profound ways. Adaptive immunity plays a central role in this dynamic. The capacity of the immune system to adapt and learn is critical in controlling parasitic infections. However, parasites continuously refine their strategies to counter these adaptations, leading to a never-ending cycle of adaptation and counter-adaptation. The evolutionary pressures imposed by this conflict have led to an extraordinary diversity of parasitic life strategies.

The future of parasitic disease research is bright, but also challenging. The need for new drugs and vaccines, particularly for those parasites resistant to current treatments, is paramount. Research into novel therapeutic strategies, such as exploring the parasite's unique biology for new drug targets, or developing vaccines, is crucial. Moreover, ongoing research into improved diagnostic methods and better understanding of disease pathogenesis will help us develop more effective control strategies and refine existing interventions. The ultimate goal is to minimize the global burden of parasitic diseases and improve the health and well-being of affected populations worldwide.

1.1 Defining Parasitism

Parasitism, at its core, is a biological interaction where one organism, the parasite, benefits at the expense of another, the host. This isn't simply a matter of one organism consuming another; it's a complex, often long-term relationship characterized by a degree of dependency. The parasite relies on the host for sustenance, shelter, and reproduction, often causing harm to the host in the process, though this harm can vary widely in severity. Some parasitic relationships are relatively benign, causing minimal damage, while others can be devastating, leading to chronic illness or even death. Understanding this spectrum of harm is crucial to grasping the nature of parasitism. The key differentiator between parasitism and predation lies in the duration of the relationship. Predators typically kill and consume their prey relatively quickly. Parasites, conversely, maintain a prolonged association with their host, often throughout their entire lifecycle or a significant portion thereof. This extended interaction allows for the evolution of sophisticated adaptations on both the parasite's and host's sides, resulting in a constant evolutionary arms race. The co-evolutionary dynamics are intricate and often involve trade-offs and compromises between parasite virulence and host resistance. Parasite survival hinges on balancing the need to extract resources from the host with the risk of killing the host prematurely, thus ending its own lifeline.

Defining parasitism also necessitates differentiating it from commensalism and mutualism. In commensalism, one organism benefits while the other is neither harmed nor benefited. A classic example is the relationship between certain bacteria and humans, where the bacteria find a home in our bodies without significantly impacting our health. Mutualism, on the other hand, describes an interaction where both organisms benefit, such as the symbiotic relationship between some plants and mycorrhizal fungi. Parasitism, however, is distinctly characterized by the net negative impact on the host, making it a unique and often detrimental form of biological interaction.

The degree of harm caused by a parasite is not static, but rather a dynamic process influenced by numerous factors. These include the parasite's virulence, the host's immune response, the environment, and the overall health status of the host. A highly virulent parasite in a weakened host will likely cause more significant damage than a less virulent parasite in a healthy host. This highlights the importance of considering multiple facets in understanding the consequences of parasitic infections. Even seemingly mild parasitic infections can pose serious risks, particularly in immunocompromised individuals. It's a nuanced relationship which varies widely across species, environments, and even individual interactions.

The study of parasitism extends beyond a simple dichotomy of parasite and host. It's a dynamic field encompassing intricate interactions and complex evolutionary trajectories. The parasites themselves show remarkable diversity in their biology, life cycles, and the strategies they utilize to survive and reproduce. Understanding this diversity is essential for developing effective prevention and treatment strategies, as each parasite demands a nuanced and targeted approach. Effective parasitic disease management depends heavily on this detailed knowledge. Moreover, advancements in molecular biology and genomics have opened up new avenues for investigating the intricacies of host-parasite interactions. The future of parasitology looks toward deeper understanding of these relationships, helping in tackling challenging diseases which plague large portions of the human population. The potential for new interventions and treatments is immense.

1.2 Parasite Diversity

The sheer variety of parasitic organisms is astounding. From the microscopic single-celled Plasmodium falciparum, the causative agent of malaria, to the macroscopic tapeworms that can reach several meters in length, the spectrum of parasitic life is breathtaking in its scope. This diversity reflects a remarkable array of adaptations honed over millennia of coevolution with their respective hosts. This complexity underscores the challenges in understanding and treating parasitic diseases, a task demanding a deep appreciation for the specific characteristics of each parasite.

Understanding this diversity isn't simply an academic exercise; it's crucial for effective diagnosis and treatment. Consider, for instance, the differences between intestinal nematodes like hookworms and the blood-borne trypanosomes that cause sleeping sickness. Their life cycles, the tissues they infect, and the resulting pathologies are vastly different, necessitating distinct diagnostic and therapeutic approaches. A generalized treatment strategy would be ineffective, even potentially harmful, given the unique characteristics of each parasite.

Moreover, this diversity extends beyond simply their morphology and life cycles. The mechanisms by which these organisms evade the host immune system also vary significantly. Some parasites employ antigenic variation, constantly changing their surface proteins to avoid detection by immune cells, while others actively suppress the host's immune response, creating an environment conducive to their survival and proliferation. These different evasion strategies further complicate treatment and highlight the need for tailored interventions.

Many parasites exhibit remarkable plasticity in their life cycle, often involving complex transformations and intermediate hosts. This complexity makes understanding their transmission dynamics and developing effective control measures particularly challenging. Take Toxoplasma gondii as an example, a protozoan parasite with a complex life cycle involving both cats and intermediate hosts like rodents and humans. Its ability to form cysts in various tissues further complicates control efforts and underscores the difficulty of eliminating the parasite completely.

The diversity of parasites is not merely a matter of species richness; it also encompasses the vast range of hosts they can infect. Some parasites are highly specialized, infecting only one or a few closely related species. Others, like Entamoeba histolytica, the causative agent of amoebic dysentery, exhibit a broader host range, impacting humans and various other mammals. This variability in host specificity influences the transmission dynamics and the epidemiology of parasitic infections, making generalized control measures difficult to implement.

Geographical distribution also plays a significant role in parasite diversity. Tropical and subtropical regions often harbor a higher diversity of parasites, reflecting factors like climate, vector availability, and human population density. Understanding these geographical patterns is crucial for designing effective prevention and control strategies, focusing resources on regions with the highest disease burden and the greatest diversity of pathogenic species.

Furthermore, the impact of parasitic infections varies significantly depending on the host's age, nutritional status, and underlying health conditions. Immunocompromised individuals, for example, are particularly susceptible to severe parasitic infections. Understanding these host factors is critical in predicting disease severity and in personalizing treatment strategies. This highlights the importance of a holistic approach, considering not only the parasite but also the host's overall health and environmental context.

Finally, and perhaps most importantly, the study of parasitic diversity is essential for understanding the evolutionary arms race between parasites and their hosts. This ongoing struggle has driven the development of remarkable adaptations in both parasites and their hosts, shaping their respective immune systems and life histories. Analyzing these adaptations provides valuable insights into the fundamental processes of evolution and natural selection. This evolutionary perspective is not only intrinsically interesting, but also fundamentally important for predicting parasite evolution and developing effective control measures in the future.

2 Cellular Invasion Mechanisms

Many parasites employ active penetration, forcefully entering host cells. Imagine a tiny spearhead, a parasite's specialized structure, piercing the cell membrane. This often involves enzymatic activity, weakening the cell's defenses. The parasite may secrete enzymes that degrade the extracellular matrix, a scaffold surrounding cells, creating an opening. This active process requires energy and sophisticated mechanisms, showcasing the parasite's remarkable adaptation. Specific examples include Toxoplasma gondii, which uses its apical complex to invade host cells, and Entamoeba histolytica, which employs a combination of mechanical force and enzymatic activity to penetrate the intestinal lining. Understanding these mechanisms is crucial for developing targeted therapies.

Passive entry, in contrast, relies on exploiting existing pathways or vulnerabilities within the host. Parasites might hitch a ride on phagocytic cells, immune cells designed to engulf foreign particles, cleverly hiding within. They may also enter through wounds or damaged tissues, taking advantage of compromised defenses. This strategy is often less energy-intensive for the parasite but depends on the host's state and susceptibility. Think of the opportunistic nature of many bacterial infections; similar principles apply to certain parasitic entries. Understanding the specific vulnerabilities used by the parasite is critical for preventative strategies like improved sanitation and wound care.

Cellular hijacking, a more insidious strategy, involves manipulation of the host cell's machinery. The parasite doesn't just invade; it takes control, reprogramming the cell to its own benefit. This can include altering gene expression, modifying cellular transport pathways, or even inducing apoptosis (programmed cell death) in surrounding cells to create a more hospitable environment. The parasite essentially becomes a puppeteer, controlling the host cell's functions for its survival and replication. Examples include the manipulation of host cell cytoskeletal elements to facilitate intracellular movement and the subversion of host immune responses to avoid detection. This sophisticated manipulation requires a deep understanding of host-parasite interactions and cellular processes.

Some parasites cleverly disguise themselves, masking their identity from the host's immune system. This "molecular camouflage" might involve mimicking host molecules or rapidly changing their surface proteins, making them difficult to recognize. Others produce molecules that actively suppress the immune response, creating a sanctuary in the host's body. This is an evolutionary arms race, with parasites continuously developing new ways to evade detection and the host's immune system adapting to counter these strategies. A classic example is the antigenic variation observed in trypanosomes, causing African sleeping sickness. These constant changes present significant challenges for vaccine development.

The success of a parasite's invasion is often determined by its ability to overcome these host defenses. This intricate interplay of strategies—active penetration, passive entry, and cellular hijacking—highlights the evolutionary sophistication of parasitic organisms and the constant challenge they present to their hosts. A thorough understanding of these mechanisms is paramount for developing effective therapeutic strategies, highlighting the need for innovative approaches to combating parasitic diseases. Ultimately, effective treatments might target specific molecules or pathways involved in invasion, preventing the parasite from gaining a foothold within the host. Further research into the molecular details of these mechanisms is crucial for future advancements in parasitology. This understanding informs the development of new drugs and preventative measures. It underscores the importance of interdisciplinary approaches, combining parasitology, immunology, and cell biology, to tackle the complex challenge of parasitic disease.

2.1 Active Penetration

Active penetration, a forceful invasion, is a hallmark strategy employed by several parasitic species. Unlike passive entry, which relies on exploiting pre-existing weaknesses in host defenses, active penetration involves the parasite directly breaching cellular barriers. This process often necessitates specialized structures and mechanisms, reflecting the parasite's remarkable adaptation for survival. Consider the Trypanosoma cruzi, the causative agent of Chagas disease. This kinetoplastid protozoan employs a unique mechanism: it actively penetrates host cells, including cardiac muscle cells, through a process involving the parasite's own motility and the secretion of lytic enzymes. These enzymes weaken the cell membrane, facilitating entry. The parasite's flagellum propels it forward, effectively drilling its way into the host cell. The resulting infection can lead to significant cardiac complications.

The exact molecular mechanisms underpinning active penetration are complex and often species-specific. However, several common themes emerge. Many actively penetrating parasites utilize specialized secretory organelles containing a cocktail of hydrolytic enzymes, such as proteases and lipases. These enzymes degrade components of the host cell membrane and extracellular matrix, creating pathways for entry. The parasite then utilizes its own cytoskeletal components and motor proteins to physically force its way into the cell.

Some parasites, like certain species of Entamoeba, release cysteine proteases that facilitate penetration through the intestinal mucosa. The resulting damage can cause inflammation and diarrhea, symptomatic of amoebiasis.

Furthermore, the host cell itself plays a significant role. The cellular response to the invading parasite can influence the success of the penetration process. For example, the composition and integrity of the host cell membrane, as well as the activity of its repair mechanisms, influence the parasite's ability to breach the cell. Factors such as the host's immune status can also affect the outcome. A compromised immune system may be less effective at containing the infection, allowing for more successful parasite penetration. Studying the interplay between the parasite's offensive strategies and the host's defensive mechanisms provides crucial insight into the pathogenesis of parasitic diseases.

For instance, Plasmodium falciparum, the most virulent species causing malaria, exhibits a complex active penetration mechanism to infect red blood cells. This involves the parasite's apical complex, a specialized structure containing proteins crucial for cell invasion. These proteins bind to specific receptors on the red blood cell surface, initiating the invasion process. Simultaneously, the parasite releases molecules that modulate the host cell membrane, aiding penetration. This targeted and multi-step invasion process highlights the sophistication of parasitic strategies to overcome host defenses.

Consequently, understanding these mechanisms is vital in developing novel anti-malarial drugs that target specific components of the invasion machinery.

In contrast to the often forceful nature of active penetration, some parasites have evolved more subtle strategies to achieve cellular entry. The mechanism can involve the exploitation of existing host cell processes, such as endocytosis or phagocytosis. These pathways, typically involved in cellular uptake of nutrients or debris, are subverted by the parasite to facilitate its entry. The parasite cleverly mimics host molecules, or even delivers signaling molecules, that trigger the host cell to engulf it. This deceptive approach allows the parasite to circumvent the physical barriers and gain entry without significant cellular damage. The successful execution of such mechanisms is critical to the pathogenicity of certain parasites.

The research into parasite penetration is not merely academic. It has direct implications for therapeutic interventions. A deep understanding of the molecular mechanisms involved in active penetration opens avenues for developing targeted therapies. These therapies could focus on inhibiting the key enzymes involved in the degradation of host cell components, interfering with the parasite's motility, or blocking the parasite's ability to bind to host cell receptors. Furthermore, research continues to explore the possibility of developing drugs that modulate the host cell's response to parasitic invasion, making the host cell less susceptible to penetration. These approaches represent a shift away from broad-spectrum antiparasitic drugs, towards more targeted therapies with fewer side effects. This precision approach is crucial in combatting drug resistance, a growing concern in the field of parasitic disease treatment.

Ultimately, the study of active penetration reveals the remarkable adaptability and evolutionary prowess of parasites. These organisms have evolved sophisticated strategies to overcome host defenses and successfully invade host cells, contributing to their immense success as pathogens. By understanding the intricacies of active penetration, we can develop more effective diagnostic tools, design improved therapies, and ultimately reduce the global burden of parasitic diseases. The ongoing research in this area promises to yield significant advancements in our understanding of parasitic infections, enabling the development of innovative approaches to diagnosis and treatment. Furthermore, this knowledge enhances our ability to predict and control outbreaks, contributing to public health strategies and initiatives.

2.2 Passive Entry

Passive entry, unlike the forceful penetration detailed in the previous chapter, relies on exploiting pre-existing vulnerabilities within the host's cellular landscape. It's a subtle strategy, often involving the exploitation of natural cellular processes or weaknesses in the host's defenses. This can range from taking advantage of damaged or compromised cell membranes to utilizing specific receptor proteins on the host cell surface as points of entry. Understanding these mechanisms is crucial for developing effective preventative and therapeutic strategies.

The most common example of passive entry involves the uptake of parasites through phagocytosis, a process where cells engulf larger particles. Some parasites, such as certain protozoa, have evolved surface molecules that mimic the host's own cellular components. This clever mimicry allows them to avoid recognition by the immune system and be unknowingly engulfed by phagocytes, thus gaining access to the cellular interior. Once inside, these parasites often subvert the normal functions of the phagocytic cell, turning it into a safe haven and replication site, instead of being destroyed as intended.

Another route of passive entry involves exploiting compromised epithelial barriers. Damage to the skin or mucous membranes, whether through injury or pre-existing conditions, can create points of entry for parasites. This damage can disrupt the integrity of the epithelial layer, allowing parasites to penetrate more easily. These breaches are often exploited by parasites which might otherwise struggle to actively breach the robust barrier provided by healthy tissue. The parasite then takes advantage of the weakened defense system, initiating infection.

Furthermore, some parasites cleverly exploit specific cellular transport mechanisms. This means utilizing the processes that typically transport nutrients or other materials into the host cell. By mimicking the structures or signals necessary for these pathways, the parasite can bypass the cellular defenses and gain entry. This is a highly sophisticated method, requiring a detailed understanding of the host cell's internal functions to successfully execute. The parasite manipulates these processes, essentially using the cellular machinery against the host.

The study of passive entry often involves intricate investigations into receptor-ligand interactions. The parasite may possess surface molecules, or ligands, that specifically bind to receptors on the host cell surface. This binding initiates a cascade of events, leading to cellular internalization of the parasite. Such investigations require advanced techniques such as flow cytometry and confocal microscopy to visualize and quantify these interactions. These methods allow researchers to elucidate the specific molecular mechanisms involved and to identify potential drug targets that could disrupt the parasite's entry.

Moreover, understanding the specifics of passive entry is not just academically interesting; it holds immense practical implications. Developing strategies to prevent passive entry requires a focus on strengthening host defenses. This could involve identifying ways to maintain the integrity of epithelial barriers, enhancing immune surveillance, or even targeting the specific receptors that parasites utilize for entry. By understanding the passive entry strategies of various parasites, we can better develop targeted therapies to disrupt this process and prevent infection. This could involve developing drugs that block the binding of parasite ligands to host receptors, or drugs that strengthen cellular barriers and the immune system. The impact of such research is clear: effective prevention is far superior to treatment.

In the case of certain parasites, the initial passive entry is just the beginning of a complex process of cellular manipulation and hijacking, a topic that will be explored in more detail in a subsequent chapter. The importance of understanding passive entry cannot be overstated, as many parasitic infections begin with this seemingly inconspicuous method of invasion. Preventing this initial step is key to preventing the disease that often follows. Therefore, the research surrounding this type of infection remains a crucial area of study within medical parasitology, particularly for the identification of new preventative strategies and treatments. Studying passive entry allows us to better understand the dynamics of the host-parasite relationship and the complex interplay between parasite strategies and the host's response. It's a subtle but significant battleground in the fight against parasitic diseases. The ongoing research promises to provide new insight and improved ways to fight these often debilitating infections. The long-term impact of such research may well revolutionize the way we prevent and treat parasitic diseases.

2.3 Cellular Hijacking

Many parasites don't simply enter cells; they commandeer them, transforming the host cell into a parasite-producing factory. This process, known as cellular hijacking, involves a complex interplay of parasite molecules and host cell machinery. Understanding these intricate molecular mechanisms is crucial for developing effective therapeutic strategies. For example, Toxoplasma gondii, a ubiquitous protozoan parasite, expertly manipulates host cell signaling pathways to promote its own replication and survival. It achieves this by secreting effector proteins that interact with host proteins, altering their functions to facilitate parasite entry and replication within the host cell. This results in the formation of a parasitophorous vacuole, a membrane-bound compartment within the host cell, which protects the parasite from the host's immune system. The parasite then uses the host cell's resources to replicate, eventually leading to cell lysis and the release of numerous daughter parasites, initiating a new round of infection. The manipulation is incredibly specific, targeting essential host cellular processes, demonstrating a remarkable level of parasite sophistication.

Unlike passive entry, where parasites rely on host cell processes for internalization, active hijacking is a more aggressive strategy involving the active modulation of host cellular mechanisms. This involves the parasite injecting proteins into the host cell, manipulating its cytoskeleton, and interfering with its normal functions. This often entails alterations in the cell's signaling pathways, potentially triggering uncontrolled growth and replication. Consider the case of Plasmodium falciparum, the parasite responsible for the deadliest form of malaria. This parasite exhibits advanced cellular hijacking strategies, including the evasion of cellular destruction through the modification of host erythrocyte membranes. The parasite's ability to actively remodel the host cell's surface proteins is a remarkable example of its parasitic prowess. These alterations help the parasite evade recognition and destruction by the host's immune system, leading to persistent infection and severe disease. Such detailed knowledge of how Plasmodium interacts with the host cell is pivotal in the development of effective antimalarial drugs.

The consequences of cellular hijacking extend beyond mere replication. Parasites can alter host cell metabolism, gene expression, and even the cell's morphology. This leads to a wide array of symptoms, depending on the specific parasite and the host cell type affected. For example, some parasites induce significant changes in host cell morphology, leading to the formation of distinctive structures that are characteristic of particular infections. These changes are not merely cosmetic; they can severely impair the host cell's function and contribute significantly to the overall pathology of the disease. Moreover, certain parasites can reprogram the host cell's metabolism to produce molecules that benefit the parasite. This metabolic redirection can result in the depletion of essential nutrients for the host cell, further weakening the host's immune response. The subtle and not-so-subtle manipulations performed by parasites are astonishingly sophisticated.

Effective treatment strategies require a thorough understanding of these intricate processes. Targeting the parasite's effector proteins, the specific host proteins they interact with, or the signaling pathways involved in hijacking could represent novel therapeutic approaches. The development of drugs that block parasite entry, inhibit parasite replication, or reverse the changes induced by hijacking are active areas of research. For instance, investigations into specific pathways manipulated by the parasite within the host cell can offer crucial insights for developing targeted therapies. Research into effective inhibitors of these pathways offers potential for new, more effective treatments that minimize side effects. This involves designing drugs that selectively disrupt the parasite's ability to manipulate the host cell without harming the host's own cells.

The study of cellular hijacking isn't just about treating existing infections; it also holds crucial insights into fundamental cellular biology. By understanding how parasites manipulate host cells, we can gain a deeper understanding of the normal functioning of our own cells. The intricate mechanisms employed by parasites often highlight fundamental cellular processes, offering unique perspectives on how cells interact, communicate, and respond to various stimuli. This knowledge might not only lead to effective treatments for parasitic infections but also contribute to our understanding of other diseases. For example, uncovering specific mechanisms by which a parasite manipulates signaling pathways can illuminate similar mechanisms in human diseases unrelated to parasitism. Ultimately, studying cellular hijacking allows us to see how cellular processes can be hijacked, offering insight into cancer and other dysfunctions. This approach can also offer a unique perspective on host-pathogen interactions.

3 Immune Evasion Strategies

Many parasites, particularly those causing chronic infections, have evolved incredibly effective ways to avoid detection and destruction by the human immune system. This evasion is crucial for their survival and propagation. These strategies aren't just single mechanisms; they're often a complex interplay of multiple tactics, creating a formidable defense against our immune response.

Antigenic variation is a prime example of this sophisticated evasion. Imagine a parasite constantly changing its "clothing," its surface proteins, so the immune system, having learned to recognize one "outfit," is constantly chasing a moving target. This continuous shifting of antigens prevents the formation of a lasting, protective immune response. Many pathogens, like the malaria parasite Plasmodium falciparum, master this technique, presenting numerous variations of their surface proteins, making it extremely difficult for our immune system to keep up. This constant change is a key factor in malaria's persistence, despite our best efforts at control and eradication.

Another crucial immune evasion strategy involves direct suppression of the host immune system. This isn't simply a matter of hiding; it's actively hindering the immune response's effectiveness. Some parasites achieve this by interfering with the signaling pathways that coordinate the immune response. They may produce molecules that suppress the activity of immune cells, like T cells or macrophages, preventing them from attacking the parasite effectively. Others may even directly target the production of cytokines, the signaling molecules that regulate the immune system, thus dampening the overall response. The impact is a weakened immune system, vulnerable not only to the parasite but also to secondary infections.

Consider the impact on the host. Immune suppression, while necessary for parasite survival, often leads to significant problems for the infected individual. This weakened immune state is the gateway to secondary infections, opportunistic pathogens that wouldn't normally pose a threat gaining a foothold. Weakened immune systems can also increase the severity and duration of the parasitic infection itself. The parasite is not only able to survive but to thrive, potentially leading to chronic illness and considerable health risks for the host.

Beyond these direct mechanisms, some parasites adopt more indirect approaches to immune evasion. They might manipulate the host's immune cells, effectively turning them into allies rather than adversaries. This Trojan horse approach is remarkably effective. For example, some parasites can enter immune cells, using them as a means of transport or as a protected haven from the immune system's scrutiny. This intracellular refuge allows the parasites to evade detection and replication, potentially undetected, allowing them to multiply within the protected environment of an immune cell itself. Furthermore, some parasites thrive in locations where the immune system's reach is limited. These microenvironments, often privileged sites shielded from immune surveillance, provide a safe haven for the parasite. This can be as simple as inhabiting areas with limited immune cell access, such as the brain or the eye, or creating enclosed environments within the host's tissues, creating a sort of protective cocoon. Here, the immune system's effectiveness is reduced. Their ability to evade the immune response in these protected niches explains why some parasitic infections are so persistent and challenging to treat.

The complexity and diversity of immune evasion strategies highlight the remarkable evolutionary adaptations of parasites. These are not random events; they are the result of millions of years of co-evolution with their hosts. Understanding these complex mechanisms is vital for developing effective treatments and preventive strategies. The strategies are often finely tuned to target specific aspects of the immune system, showcasing the intricate interplay between parasite and host.

The implications for developing effective treatments are clear. Traditional approaches that simply aim to eliminate the parasite may prove inadequate if the parasite's immune evasion strategies remain intact. A comprehensive understanding of these mechanisms is essential for the development of new treatments that could target these immune evasion mechanisms directly, rather than simply focusing on parasite eradication. We need treatments that work on multiple fronts. Treatments might focus on enhancing the host's immune response, thereby improving the ability to combat the infection, or on interfering with the parasite's ability to suppress the immune system, restoring the host's defenses. Ultimately, this improved understanding can lead to more effective therapies and better strategies to combat these persistent and devastating infections.

Finally, future research should focus on further elucidating the molecular mechanisms underpinning these immune evasion strategies. Detailed knowledge of the specific molecules and pathways involved will pave the way for the development of novel therapeutic interventions and vaccines. Targeting these specific components might be far more effective than broadly targeting the parasite itself. This nuanced approach will be key to developing more effective control and prevention strategies for parasitic infections worldwide. The complexity of parasite immune evasion presents a substantial challenge, yet simultaneously offers promising avenues for innovation in therapeutic approaches to parasitic infections.

3.1 Antigenic Variation

Antigenic variation is a crucial survival strategy employed by many parasites to evade the host's immune system. This remarkable ability allows them to constantly change their surface proteins, effectively rendering previously generated antibodies useless. Imagine a game of cat and mouse, where the mouse (parasite) is constantly changing its coat to avoid detection by the cat (immune system). This continuous molecular disguise is paramount to their persistent infection. Understanding this process is key to developing effective long-term treatments.

The mechanism behind antigenic variation is complex and varies across different parasite species. Some parasites achieve this through gene rearrangement, essentially shuffling their genetic deck to produce a new surface protein. Others use a "switch" mechanism, turning on and off different genes that encode for surface antigens. Think of it as a sophisticated wardrobe, where the parasite selects different "outfits" (antigens) depending on the immune pressure it faces. This dynamic interplay between parasite and host is a fascinating aspect of the evolutionary arms race.

Consider Trypanosoma brucei, the parasite responsible for African trypanosomiasis (sleeping sickness). This protozoan masterfully utilizes antigenic variation to evade the host's immune response. It expresses a vast repertoire of variant surface glycoproteins (VSGs), which are constantly switched, allowing it to avoid immune detection for prolonged periods. This extended evasion allows chronic infection, leading to the debilitating symptoms of the disease. The sheer number of potential VSGs is staggering, making it extremely difficult for the immune system to keep up. Each VSG is encoded by a separate gene, and the parasite selects which gene to express.

In contrast, some parasites, such as Plasmodium falciparum, the causative agent of malaria, employ a different approach. While they do not have the same extensive VSG repertoire as Trypanosoma brucei, they still exhibit antigenic variation through other mechanisms. They manipulate the expression of various surface proteins, subtly altering their antigenicity. This subtle shift can still be sufficient to delay or evade immune recognition. The timing and pattern of this variation are often complex, potentially influenced by factors like the host's immune response and the parasite's developmental stage. Understanding these nuances is critical for vaccine development.

The clinical implications of antigenic variation are significant. The ability of parasites to evade the immune system contributes to persistent infections, chronic disease, and relapse. Treatment often proves challenging because the immune system's memory response is ineffective against the constantly changing surface antigens. This highlights the importance of developing therapies that target conserved parasite structures, unaffected by antigenic variation. Focusing on mechanisms independent of the variable surface antigens is essential for effective long-term disease management.

Developing effective vaccines against parasites that exhibit antigenic variation poses a significant challenge. Traditional vaccine approaches, which focus on inducing immunity against specific surface antigens, are often ineffective because the parasite can quickly change its antigenicity, rendering the vaccine useless. This problem necessitates innovative vaccine strategies that target conserved parasite molecules, those less susceptible to antigenic variation. Researchers are actively exploring alternative strategies, focusing on conserved parasite molecules, such as intracellular proteins, which are less likely to undergo change.

Further research is crucial to fully understand the mechanisms of antigenic variation across different parasite species. This involves uncovering the molecular details of gene switching, identifying the regulatory elements controlling antigen expression, and dissecting the parasite's interactions with the host's immune system. A deeper understanding of these processes will provide valuable insights for the development of novel therapeutic and preventive strategies. This is a complex but critical area of research with potentially life-saving implications. Advances in genomic sequencing, proteomics, and immunology are providing new tools to unravel the complexities of this phenomenon. In essence, tackling antigenic variation is akin to deciphering a complex code, a code that parasites use to evade our immune system and cause disease.

3.2 Immune Suppression

Immune suppression is a crucial mechanism employed by many parasites to establish and maintain infection. Successfully evading the host's immune system is paramount for their survival and propagation. This involves a complex interplay of molecular mimicry, manipulation of immune cells, and direct inhibition of immune responses. Some parasites produce molecules that actively suppress the production of pro-inflammatory cytokines, crucial signaling molecules that orchestrate the immune response. This dampening effect weakens the host's ability to effectively recognize and eliminate the parasite.

The suppression of T-cell responses is another commonly observed strategy. T cells, a vital component of the adaptive immune system, are responsible for targeted destruction of infected cells. Parasites, through various mechanisms, can interfere with T-cell activation, proliferation, and differentiation, effectively rendering them less potent in combating the infection. This manipulation can involve the secretion of immunosuppressive molecules that directly inhibit T-cell activity or indirectly disrupt the signaling pathways involved in their activation. This often leads to a prolonged infection and the persistence of the parasite within the host.

Moreover, parasites often target other key players in the immune system, including B cells and natural killer (NK) cells. B cells are responsible for the production of antibodies, which are essential for recognizing and neutralizing pathogens. Parasites can circumvent antibody-mediated immunity by altering their surface antigens, thereby avoiding recognition and binding by antibodies. Similarly, NK cells, crucial for early innate immune responses, can be suppressed by parasites, further contributing to the weakening of the host's immune defense. These strategies demonstrate remarkable sophistication in manipulating the host's defense mechanisms.

The degree of immune suppression varies greatly among different parasitic species and is often related to their life cycle and pathogenesis. Some parasites cause a relatively mild immune suppression, leading to a chronic but manageable infection. Others induce profound immunosuppression, resulting in severe disease and even death. Understanding the specific mechanisms of immune suppression employed by different parasites is essential for developing targeted therapies. This could involve blocking the immunosuppressive molecules produced by the parasites or stimulating the host's immune system to overcome the parasite's suppressive effects. In essence, effectively counteracting immune suppression is a primary goal in developing treatments for parasitic infections.

One of the most significant challenges in combating parasitic infections lies in the intricate interplay between the parasite and the host's immune system. Many parasitic infections are characterized by chronic inflammation, a prolonged immune response that can be as damaging as the infection itself. Ironically, the parasite's ability to suppress the immune system can contribute to this chronic inflammation, creating a paradoxical situation where the suppression initially allows the parasite to thrive, but the long-term consequences fuel a prolonged, harmful inflammatory response within the host. This complex interplay necessitates a nuanced approach to therapy, one that ideally not only targets the parasite directly but also addresses the consequences of the immune suppression induced by the infection. Future research needs to focus on uncovering these complex interactions.

Ultimately, the development of effective treatments necessitates a thorough understanding of the parasite's strategies for immune evasion. This includes not only characterizing the immunosuppressive molecules produced by the parasites but also elucidating the cellular and molecular mechanisms involved in the manipulation of the host's immune system. This complex dance between parasite and host demands advanced research techniques and interdisciplinary collaborations involving immunologists, parasitologists, and other relevant specialists to unravel the intricate details and pave the way for new treatments. A multi-pronged approach, combining drugs that directly target the parasite with strategies aimed at boosting the host's immune response, represents a promising path forward. This may involve novel immunotherapies designed to restore immune function and bolster the host's ability to combat the infection, thus effectively breaking the cycle of parasite-induced immune suppression. A holistic understanding of this interplay is therefore critical for the development of effective and lasting therapeutic solutions. Furthermore, it is crucial to appreciate that the host's genetic background and overall health significantly influence their response to parasitic infections. A weakened immune system, due to pre-existing conditions or malnutrition, can further exacerbate the effects of immune suppression, making the infection even more challenging to manage.

The study of immune suppression in parasitic infections is an active and evolving field. New research continues to reveal the sophisticated strategies parasites employ to evade the host's immune system. This increased understanding fuels the development of novel therapies designed to counteract these strategies and improve treatment outcomes. Ongoing research focuses on understanding the genetic basis of immune suppression, identifying new drug targets, and exploring innovative immunotherapeutic approaches. These efforts aim to provide more effective and safer treatments for parasitic infections, reducing their global health burden and improving quality of life for affected individuals. The complexity of these interactions however underscores the need for a sustained and collaborative research effort to fully unravel the mysteries of parasitic immune evasion and ultimately develop more effective therapies.

4 Disease Manifestations

Understanding the clinical presentation of parasitic infections is crucial for effective diagnosis and treatment. Symptoms vary wildly depending on the specific parasite, its location in the body, the intensity of the infection, and the individual host's immune response. For example, malaria, caused by Plasmodium species, manifests with cyclical fevers, chills, sweats, and headache. In contrast, intestinal parasites like Giardia lamblia often cause diarrhea, abdominal cramps, and bloating. The diversity in symptoms underscores the need for a comprehensive approach to diagnosis.

The underlying pathogenesis, or the biological mechanisms causing disease, is equally diverse. Many parasites directly damage host tissues through their feeding or migratory activities. Others produce toxins that disrupt cellular function or trigger inflammatory responses. Some parasites, such as schistosomes, induce granuloma formation—localized areas of inflammation—around their eggs, leading to significant organ damage. Still others, like Trypanosoma brucei, evade the immune system, leading to chronic, debilitating infections. A thorough understanding of these diverse mechanisms is essential for developing effective therapies.

Clinical presentations can range from mild, self-limiting infections to severe, life-threatening illnesses. The severity depends on several factors. The parasite's virulence, or its ability to cause disease, plays a significant role. The number of parasites infecting the host (parasite load) also influences disease severity, with higher loads generally leading to more severe symptoms. The host's nutritional status, overall health, and immune competency are also key determinants. A compromised immune system can allow an otherwise manageable infection to become severe, highlighting the interconnectedness of host factors and parasitic pathogenesis.

Accurate diagnosis requires a multifaceted approach. Microscopic examination of blood smears, stool samples, or other bodily fluids often reveals the presence of parasites or their eggs. Molecular diagnostic techniques, such as PCR, offer increased sensitivity and specificity, particularly for detecting low-level infections or identifying specific parasite species. Serological tests, detecting antibodies against the parasite, can be useful in certain cases, although they may not differentiate between active and past infections. The choice of diagnostic test depends on the suspected parasite and the clinical presentation.

Disease progression is a dynamic process, often marked by distinct stages. The initial stages may involve asymptomatic infection, with the parasite establishing itself within the host without causing noticeable symptoms. This asymptomatic phase can be prolonged, particularly in chronic infections. As the parasite burden increases or the host's immune response is compromised, the infection may progress to symptomatic stages, with the onset of characteristic clinical manifestations. In some cases, chronic infections can lead to irreversible organ damage or other long-term complications.

Consider Toxoplasma gondii, a ubiquitous parasite that can cause toxoplasmosis. In healthy individuals, infection is often asymptomatic or manifests with mild flu-like symptoms. However, in individuals with compromised immune systems, such as those with HIV/AIDS, toxoplasmosis can lead to severe encephalitis, a life-threatening brain infection. This stark difference highlights the crucial role of the host's immune status in shaping disease progression. Understanding this progression is paramount for timely intervention and effective management of parasitic infections.

The clinical picture of parasitic infections is often complex, encompassing a broad spectrum of symptoms, pathological processes, and disease courses. Precise diagnosis and understanding of the underlying mechanisms are essential for effective treatment strategies and public health interventions. The knowledge of disease manifestation in parasitic infections continues to evolve with ongoing research uncovering new insights into the host-parasite interaction and disease pathogenesis. Therefore, continuous learning and adaptation are vital for healthcare professionals working in this field. This multifaceted nature emphasizes the importance of a holistic approach to diagnosis and management, considering the interaction between parasite, host, and environment. The impact of socioeconomic factors, access to healthcare, and environmental conditions can significantly influence the outcome of parasitic infections and underscore the need for targeted public health strategies in endemic regions. Each parasitic infection presents its unique challenges, demanding a keen eye for detail and an extensive knowledge base. This chapter serves as an initial exploration of this complex realm, intending to provide a foundational understanding of the varied symptoms, pathogeneses, diagnostic tools, and disease trajectories associated with parasitic infections. Further exploration into specific parasites and their corresponding clinical manifestations is encouraged to cultivate a more detailed understanding of this intricate subject matter. Remember, the ultimate goal is not merely to diagnose, but to effectively manage and ultimately mitigate the impact of these infections. Thorough knowledge and comprehensive approaches are crucial for achieving optimal patient outcomes.

4.1 Symptoms & Signs

Recognizing the symptoms and signs of parasitic infection is crucial for timely diagnosis and effective treatment. The presentation varies greatly depending on the specific parasite, the location of the infection within the body, and the individual's immune response.

Some infections manifest with subtle, almost imperceptible symptoms, while others cause severe, life-threatening illness. Understanding this spectrum is essential for any healthcare professional dealing with suspected parasitic disease.

Fever, a common symptom across numerous parasitic infections, often indicates the body's immune response battling the invader. Its severity can range from a mild elevation to a dangerously high temperature, signaling the intensity of the infection and the host's response. Alongside fever, fatigue can be a significant indicator; a debilitating tiredness that goes beyond normal tiredness, impacting daily activities and overall well-being. This fatigue, often coupled with malaise—a general feeling of discomfort—reflects the body's struggle against the parasite.

Gastrointestinal symptoms represent another significant category of clinical manifestations. Diarrhea, ranging from mild to severe and potentially chronic, frequently accompanies intestinal parasitic infections. Abdominal pain, cramping, and bloating are other common symptoms reflecting the parasite's presence and activity in the digestive tract. Nausea and vomiting can accompany these symptoms, further hindering the body's ability to absorb nutrients and maintain hydration, adding a layer of debility to the illness. Changes in bowel habits, such as increased frequency or altered stool consistency, provide important diagnostic clues and can indicate the severity of the infection. These symptoms, though often overlooked in early stages, become critical when evaluating the overall health and progression of the disease.

Beyond the gastrointestinal system, many parasites affect other organ systems. Hepatic involvement, for instance, can manifest as jaundice (yellowing of the skin and eyes) or abnormal liver function tests. Similarly, neurological symptoms can appear in cases of parasites affecting the central nervous system. These symptoms vary and may range from mild headache and cognitive impairment to severe seizures and neurological deficits. Respiratory symptoms such as cough, shortness of breath, and wheezing are also possible, often associated with parasitic lung infections, particularly in immunocompromised individuals.

Skin manifestations can provide highly visual clues. Rashes, itching, and lesions are common signs and symptoms. The specific appearance of these skin changes is dependent on the parasitic species and the body's reaction to it, often showing unique characteristics helpful in diagnosis. Some parasites produce distinct skin lesions; their shape, size, and distribution on the body can greatly aid in identifying the causative agent.

Anemia, a decrease in red blood cells, is a common consequence of parasitic infections, often resulting from blood loss or nutritional deficiencies caused by the parasite. This can lead to fatigue, weakness, and shortness of breath, further compounding the patient's symptoms. Lymphadenopathy, or swollen lymph nodes, may indicate the body's immune response actively fighting the infection. The location and size of swollen lymph nodes can provide additional diagnostic information concerning the specific site of infection.

Diagnosing parasitic infections requires a multi-pronged approach. Physical examinations, identifying specific symptoms or skin manifestations, are essential. Stool analysis helps detect intestinal parasites and their eggs or larvae. Blood tests can detect parasitic antigens or antibodies, indicating the presence of a specific parasitic infection. Imaging techniques like ultrasound, computed tomography (CT) scans, or magnetic resonance imaging (MRI) scans might be necessary for visualizing the parasites or associated lesions. In some cases, biopsy might be needed to obtain tissue samples for microscopic examination. Each test plays a specific role, and a comprehensive approach combining several tests ensures accurate diagnosis. The diagnostic process must consider the geographical location of the patient and their travel history, as this significantly impacts the likelihood of various parasites.

It is important to emphasize that this chapter does not provide an exhaustive list. The symptoms and signs of parasitic infections are extremely varied, and this only highlights some of the most common manifestations. This information is for educational purposes, not for self-diagnosis or treatment, and always seek professional medical advice for any health concerns. Accurate diagnosis requires a complete evaluation by a healthcare professional who can appropriately interpret the presenting symptoms within the context of the patient's medical history and current health status.

4.2 Pathogenesis

Understanding the pathogenesis of parasitic diseases requires a nuanced approach, moving beyond simple cause-and-effect relationships. It's a complex interplay of parasite factors, host responses, and environmental influences. Consider, for example, Plasmodium falciparum, the causative agent of the most severe form of malaria. Its ability to successfully invade red blood cells hinges on specific interactions between parasite proteins and host cell receptors. This initial invasion isn't merely a physical breach; it's a sophisticated molecular dance, involving intricate signaling pathways and a delicate balance of adhesion molecules. The parasite's success relies not only on its own invasive mechanisms, but also on the host's susceptibility, influenced by genetics and prior exposure.

The subsequent stages of the parasite's lifecycle are equally intricate, each contributing to the overall pathogenesis. Intracellular replication within red blood cells leads to their eventual rupture, releasing merozoites and triggering a cascade of inflammatory responses. These responses, though crucial for defense, can also contribute to the severity of the disease. The inflammatory cascade, involving cytokines and chemokines, can lead to fever, anemia, and potentially life-threatening complications like cerebral malaria, where parasites obstruct blood vessels in the brain. This highlights the duality of the host response; while essential for combating the infection, an overly robust or dysregulated response can inflict significant damage.

Beyond the direct effects of parasite invasion and replication, the pathogenesis of many parasitic infections involves indirect mechanisms. Some parasites, for instance, produce toxins or metabolic byproducts that contribute to the pathology. These substances can exert a variety of effects, ranging from causing direct tissue damage to interfering with vital host processes. The specific effects depend on the parasite species and the site of infection. Consider the debilitating effects of schistosomiasis, where the eggs of the Schistosoma parasite become trapped in tissues, causing inflammation, fibrosis, and organ damage. The resulting granuloma formation, while an attempt by the host immune system to contain the infection, contributes significantly to the long-term morbidity.

Furthermore, the pathogenesis isn't a static process; it's dynamic and evolves over time. As the infection progresses, the interaction between parasite and host shifts. The initial acute phase may be characterized by intense inflammation and high parasite loads. However, chronic infections can lead to immune modulation, where the parasite manipulates the host immune system to create a more favorable environment for its survival. This can result in long-term consequences, such as immune suppression or the development of autoimmune responses. Understanding this dynamic interaction is critical for designing effective therapies. It is not a simple case of targeting the parasite alone; effective treatment strategies must also consider the host's immune response and its potential to contribute to disease severity.

The study of pathogenesis is not merely an academic exercise; it underpins the development of effective prevention and treatment strategies. By understanding the precise mechanisms involved in disease development, researchers can identify specific targets for therapeutic interventions. For instance, a detailed understanding of the molecular interactions between the malaria parasite and red blood cells has informed the development of drugs that target specific parasite proteins involved in invasion. Similarly, insights into the immune evasion strategies employed by parasites are essential for designing vaccines that can effectively stimulate protective immune responses. Therefore, the study of pathogenesis is essential not only for comprehending the complex interplay between parasite and host, but also for developing innovative approaches to control and eradicate parasitic diseases. The continual refinement of our understanding of pathogenesis remains paramount in the global fight against these infections. The development of new diagnostic tools and therapies relies on a complete and thorough knowledge of parasitic pathogenesis, from the initial invasion to the development of chronic disease. This multifaceted approach is key to developing effective treatment protocols and vaccines for a wider range of parasitic diseases. Ongoing research continues to unravel the complexities of pathogenesis, highlighting the continuous need for innovative approaches and further investigations.

4.3 Clinical Presentations

Understanding the clinical presentation of parasitic diseases is crucial for accurate diagnosis and effective treatment. The symptoms often vary widely depending on the specific parasite, the site of infection, the intensity of the infestation, and the host's immune response. Some infections may be asymptomatic, especially in individuals with robust immune systems or low parasite burdens. However, many parasitic diseases present with a broad spectrum of clinical manifestations, ranging from mild discomfort to life-threatening complications. Recognizing these diverse presentations is paramount for appropriate medical intervention.

Consider malaria, for instance. The clinical presentation of malaria, caused by Plasmodium species, can range from mild flu-like symptoms such as fever, chills, headache, and muscle aches to severe complications like cerebral malaria, acute respiratory distress syndrome, and acute kidney injury. The severity of the disease is influenced by factors such as the parasite species, the patient's age and immune status, and the presence of co-morbidities. The cyclical nature of the fever in malaria, a hallmark of the disease, is a result of the parasite's lifecycle within red blood cells. This periodic release of parasite products from lysed red blood cells triggers the characteristic febrile episodes.

Alternatively, intestinal parasitic infections, such as those caused by Giardia lamblia or Entamoeba histolytica, often manifest with gastrointestinal symptoms including diarrhea, abdominal cramps, nausea, and vomiting. The severity of these symptoms can vary greatly, with some individuals experiencing only mild discomfort while others develop severe dehydration and malnutrition. Chronic infections can lead to long-term complications such as malabsorption syndromes and weight loss. The diagnostic process often involves stool examinations to identify the parasite's cysts or trophozoites. The presence of blood or mucus in stool can suggest invasive amebiasis.

Schistosomiasis, a parasitic disease caused by Schistosoma species, presents a different clinical picture. It commonly involves skin irritation at the site of penetration by cercariae (the infective larval stage), followed by a flu-like illness. However, chronic infection can lead to a spectrum of complications affecting the liver, intestines, urinary tract, and lungs. Granulomas form around parasite eggs, leading to inflammation and tissue damage. In severe cases, portal hypertension, bladder cancer, and kidney failure can occur. Diagnostic tools such as serological tests and examination of urine or stool for parasite eggs play a crucial role in the identification of schistosomiasis.

The clinical presentation of toxoplasmosis, caused by Toxoplasma gondii, is highly dependent on the patient's immune status. In immunocompetent individuals, the infection is often asymptomatic or causes only mild flu-like symptoms. However, in individuals with compromised immune systems, such as those with HIV/AIDS, toxoplasmosis can lead to severe complications, including encephalitis, myocarditis, and pneumonitis. Pregnancy also presents a unique challenge, as congenital toxoplasmosis can result in severe neurological and ophthalmological problems in the newborn. Serological testing is widely used to diagnose toxoplasmosis, enabling the detection of antibodies against the parasite.

Finally, one must consider the influence of co-infections. It's not uncommon for individuals to be infected with multiple parasites simultaneously. This co-infection can lead to complex clinical presentations that are difficult to interpret without a thorough understanding of each parasite's individual contribution to the overall disease process. Such complexity necessitates a comprehensive diagnostic approach, combining clinical evaluation, laboratory tests, and, in some instances, imaging techniques. A thorough understanding of potential co-infections is vital for accurate diagnosis and successful treatment. This holistic approach guarantees improved patient outcomes and emphasizes the multifaceted nature of parasitic infections. Effective management requires careful attention to detail and a deep understanding of the specific characteristics of each infection.

4.4 Diagnostic Approaches

Accurate diagnosis is paramount in managing parasitic infections. Misidentification can lead to ineffective treatment and potentially life-threatening complications. Therefore, a multi-pronged approach, incorporating various diagnostic techniques, is often necessary. This multifaceted strategy ensures a comprehensive assessment, maximizing the chances of successful identification and subsequent therapeutic intervention.

Microscopic examination remains a cornerstone of parasitology diagnostics. Direct examination of fecal samples, blood smears, or tissue biopsies often reveals the presence of parasitic stages such as eggs, larvae, or adult organisms. Specific staining techniques enhance visualization, helping to differentiate between various parasite species. For instance, Giemsa staining is invaluable in identifying malaria parasites within red blood cells, its characteristic staining pattern readily distinguishing Plasmodium falciparum from other species. However, microscopic methods can be labor-intensive and require significant expertise, sensitivity varying greatly depending on the parasite's life cycle stage and the experience of the microscopist.

Molecular diagnostic techniques have revolutionized the field, offering increased sensitivity and specificity. Polymerase chain reaction (PCR) is widely employed to amplify parasite DNA or RNA, detecting even minute quantities of parasitic material. Real-time PCR allows for quantitative assessment, enabling determination of parasitic load. This technique proves especially valuable in detecting low-level infections or those with limited parasite shedding, such as certain stages of Toxoplasma gondii infection. Moreover, PCR can identify specific parasite species or genotypes, guiding treatment choices and informing epidemiological studies. The high cost and technical expertise required can limit accessibility in resource-poor settings, a crucial constraint to consider.

Serological tests detect antibodies produced by the host in response to parasitic infection. Enzyme-linked immunosorbent assays (ELISAs) and indirect fluorescent antibody tests (IFATs) are commonly used to detect specific antibodies. These methods are particularly useful in diagnosing infections with parasites that are difficult to detect directly, such as Trichinella spiralis or Trypanosoma cruzi. However, serological tests may not distinguish between past and current infections, limiting their diagnostic value in determining active disease. Cross-reactivity with other infections can also lead to false-positive results, requiring careful interpretation and often necessitating corroborating evidence from other diagnostic modalities.

Imaging techniques, such as computed tomography (CT) scans, magnetic resonance imaging (MRI), and ultrasound, can visualize parasitic cysts, granulomas, or other pathological changes associated with parasitic infections. These imaging methods are especially valuable in diagnosing tissue-invasive parasites like Echinococcus species or diagnosing the effects of parasites like Schistosoma causing significant organ damage. However, imaging is not always specific to parasitic infections, and interpretation requires experience in recognizing parasitic pathology, especially in cases mimicking other disease processes. Cost and accessibility can restrict its widespread use.

Rapid diagnostic tests (RDTs) have gained popularity, offering point-of-care diagnostics for certain parasitic infections. These tests are simple to use, relatively inexpensive, and require minimal equipment, making them ideal for resource-limited settings. Most RDTs target malaria parasites, detecting specific antigens in blood samples. While RDTs can provide rapid results, their sensitivity and specificity might be lower compared to other methods, leading to potential false positive or negative results, hence interpretation necessitates cautious consideration.

The selection of diagnostic methods depends on various factors, including the suspected parasite, the clinical presentation of the patient, the availability of resources, and the expertise of the diagnostic laboratory. Often, a combination of diagnostic approaches is required to ensure an accurate diagnosis. For example, a patient presenting with fever, headache, and splenomegaly may undergo a blood smear examination to detect malaria parasites, complemented by RDTs for immediate results and PCR to confirm species identification and quantify parasitic load. Similarly, a suspected case of intestinal parasitism may involve microscopic examination of stool samples, possibly enhanced by antigen detection techniques and molecular methods if necessary. A holistic approach, considering the clinical context and integrating the strengths of different techniques, stands as the most effective path toward timely and accurate diagnosis of parasitic infections.

4.5 Disease Progression

Understanding the progression of parasitic diseases is crucial for effective diagnosis and treatment. It's not a simple linear path; instead, it's a complex interplay between the parasite's life cycle, its virulence, and the host's immune response. Factors like the initial inoculum size, the parasite's genetic makeup, and the host's nutritional status and overall health significantly influence the disease trajectory. For example, a larger inoculum of Plasmodium falciparum (the parasite that causes malaria) can lead to a more severe and rapid disease onset compared to a smaller inoculum, highlighting the importance of early diagnosis and intervention.

The initial phase, often asymptomatic or characterized by mild, nonspecific symptoms, is the insidious period of infection. During this incubation period, the parasite establishes itself within the host, multiplying and possibly evading the initial immune response. The duration of this phase varies considerably depending on the specific parasite species and the host's immune competence. Some parasites may have a relatively short incubation period, whereas others may remain dormant for extended periods, leading to chronic, relapsing infections. This highlights the challenge in early detection, as symptoms are often masked or attributed to other ailments.

The next stage often involves the emergence of more specific and pronounced symptoms. This coincides with the parasite's active replication and spread throughout the body. For instance, in malaria, this phase is marked by cyclical fever, chills, and sweats, reflecting the parasite's synchronized erythrocytic cycle. In other parasitic infections, symptoms may involve gastrointestinal disturbances, such as diarrhea and abdominal pain (e.g., giardiasis), or neurological manifestations, like encephalitis or meningitis (e.g., toxoplasmosis). The intensity and nature of these symptoms depend on the parasitic species, the location of infection, and the host's individual immune response.

As the infection progresses, the disease may enter a chronic phase, where the parasite and host reach a state of dynamic equilibrium. In some cases, this can result in a relatively asymptomatic state, with the parasite persisting at low levels within the host. However, this chronic phase can also be characterized by persistent or recurrent symptoms, potentially leading to significant morbidity and long-term health complications. For instance, chronic schistosomiasis can cause liver damage and bladder cancer. This long-term effect underscores the importance of prompt treatment, even in cases where symptoms appear mild or manageable.

The severity of the disease also depends on the parasite's ability to evade the host's immune system. Parasites have evolved sophisticated mechanisms to suppress or modulate the immune response, promoting their survival and replication. This immune evasion can be a significant factor contributing to the progression from an acute to a chronic infection. The host's genetic background, nutritional status, and pre-existing health conditions also influence the immune response and the overall course of the disease. Understanding these intricate interactions between parasite and host is pivotal for developing effective therapies and preventing long-term complications. Effective immune responses can result in parasite clearance, while weak responses may result in chronic infection and consequent morbidity.

Finally, the terminal phase can result in severe complications and even death, especially in the absence of appropriate treatment. Organ failure, severe anemia, or disseminated intravascular coagulation are some possible severe outcomes. The likelihood of reaching this stage is greatly influenced by factors like the parasite's virulence, the host's overall health, and access to healthcare. Therefore, early diagnosis and appropriate management of parasitic infections are essential to prevent adverse outcomes. This highlights the need for public health initiatives focused on prevention, early diagnosis, and access to effective treatments. The complexities in disease progression emphasize the need for comprehensive research and improved diagnostic tools.

5 Therapeutic Interventions

Effective treatment of parasitic infections requires a multifaceted approach, tailored to the specific parasite and the patient's overall health. Simple infections, often diagnosed through microscopic examination of stool or blood samples, may respond well to readily available medications. However, more complex cases, especially those involving immunocompromised individuals or those with severe infections, necessitate a more involved treatment strategy. This may involve a combination of drugs, supportive care, and close monitoring of the patient's response. Regular follow-up appointments are crucial to assess treatment efficacy and to adjust the approach as needed.

Many parasitic infections are treated with antiparasitic drugs. These drugs target various aspects of the parasite's life cycle, aiming to disrupt its metabolic processes, inhibit reproduction, or directly kill the parasite. The choice of drug depends on factors such as the type of parasite, the severity of the infection, the patient's age and health status, and potential drug interactions. Some antiparasitic drugs are broad-spectrum, effective against a variety of parasites, while others are specific to particular species.

Malaria, a parasitic disease caused by Plasmodium species, represents a significant global health challenge. Antimalarial drugs, a class of medications specifically designed to combat malaria, are crucial in managing this disease. These drugs vary in their mechanisms of action, some targeting the parasite's metabolic pathways, others interfering with its ability to replicate or invade red blood cells. The selection of antimalarial drugs is influenced by the specific Plasmodium species involved, the geographical location (due to drug resistance patterns), and the patient's condition. Treatment often involves a combination of drugs to maximize efficacy and minimize the development of resistance.

Beyond malaria, numerous other parasites infect humans, each requiring its own tailored treatment approach. Intestinal parasites, like hookworms or roundworms, may be treated with anthelmintics, medications that specifically target helminths (worms). These drugs can paralyze or kill the worms, facilitating their expulsion from the body. Protozoan infections, such as giardiasis or amoebiasis, often require different classes of antiparasitic drugs, each targeting specific aspects of the parasite's biology. The precise drug choice will often hinge on the parasite species involved, its location in the body, and any co-occurring infections or complications.

Effective treatment necessitates a nuanced understanding of the parasite's life cycle and its interaction with the host immune system. For instance, some parasites reside within red blood cells, requiring drugs capable of penetrating this cellular barrier. Others may evade the immune system, demanding a treatment strategy that supports the host's immune response. A thorough understanding of the pathogenesis of the infection is critical for choosing the most appropriate therapeutic intervention.

In certain instances, surgical intervention might be necessary. This is particularly relevant for parasitic infections causing significant tissue damage or obstruction. For example, the surgical removal of adult worms or cysts may be needed in cases of severe infection. In such instances, surgical intervention provides a vital complement to drug therapy, helping to alleviate symptoms and prevent further complications. Post-surgical care frequently includes antiparasitic medication to eliminate any remaining parasites or to treat any persistent infections. The decision to opt for surgery is made on a case-by-case basis, taking into account the severity of the infection, the patient's overall health, and the potential risks and benefits of the procedure.

Drug resistance poses a considerable threat to effective parasitic infection control. The widespread use of antiparasitic drugs has selected for resistant parasite strains, reducing the effectiveness of previously reliable treatments. Combating drug resistance requires a multi-pronged strategy, including responsible drug use, the development of new drugs with novel mechanisms of action, and the implementation of robust surveillance programs to monitor the emergence and spread of resistant strains. This collaborative approach, involving healthcare professionals, researchers, and public health officials, is crucial in ensuring that therapeutic interventions remain effective.

Beyond medication, supportive care plays a vital role in managing parasitic infections. This encompasses measures such as adequate nutrition, hydration, and pain management. Supportive care aims to maintain the patient's overall well-being and enhance their ability to recover from the infection. In cases of severe infections, supportive care may involve hospitalization to provide intensive monitoring and treatment. This includes the management of complications, such as dehydration or anemia, which can arise during the course of infection.

The development of new antiparasitic drugs remains a high priority for researchers and pharmaceutical companies. This pursuit involves the screening of novel compounds, investigating new drug targets within the parasite, and exploring new drug delivery systems. The ultimate aim is to develop drugs that are more effective, safer, and less prone to inducing resistance. This ongoing endeavor is crucial for overcoming the challenges posed by drug resistance and ensuring the continued effectiveness of therapeutic interventions against parasitic infections.

Research continues to reveal new insights into the complexities of parasite biology and host-parasite interactions. This improved understanding forms the bedrock for more targeted and effective therapeutic strategies. The use of advanced technologies such as genomics and proteomics facilitates the identification of new drug targets, while innovative approaches such as immunotherapy show promise in boosting the host's immune response. Continued investment in research and development is essential for the ongoing advancement of therapeutic interventions against these challenging infections.

5.1 Antimalarial Drugs

Malaria, a disease caused by Plasmodium parasites transmitted via mosquito bites, remains a significant global health concern. Effective treatment hinges on the judicious use of antimalarial drugs, a diverse group with varying mechanisms of action and efficacy profiles. Understanding these drugs is crucial for clinicians and public health officials alike.

Chloroquine, once a mainstay, has suffered from widespread parasite resistance, limiting its current applicability. Its mechanism involves inhibiting the parasite's heme detoxification pathway, leading to the accumulation of toxic heme and parasite death. However, the emergence of chloroquine-resistant strains significantly restricts its use, making it largely ineffective in many regions. This underscores the ever-evolving nature of the fight against malaria.

Quinine, a naturally occurring alkaloid, holds historical significance but also faces limitations due to toxicity and resistance. Its mechanism, similar to chloroquine, involves interfering with heme polymerization within the parasite. While still used in some contexts, its efficacy is often overshadowed by newer, more potent drugs and its side-effect profile necessitates careful monitoring. The challenge lies in balancing therapeutic benefit against potential adverse effects.

Artemisinin-based combination therapies (ACTs) are currently recommended as first-line treatment for uncomplicated malaria. Artemisinin derivatives, such as artesunate and artemether, possess rapid-acting properties, targeting various stages of the parasite's life cycle. The combination approach aims to mitigate the development of resistance and enhance overall efficacy. The World Health Organization (WHO) strongly advocates for ACTs due to their effectiveness and the strategy to limit resistance development.

Mefloquine, a quinoline derivative, acts on parasite mitochondria, disrupting their function. It's commonly used in prophylaxis and treatment, especially in areas with chloroquine resistance. However, neuropsychiatric side effects can limit its usability in certain populations, requiring careful consideration before prescribing, especially for those with a history of psychiatric conditions. Thorough patient assessment and informed consent are vital here.

Other antimalarials, including atovaquone-proguanil, sulfadoxine-pyrimethamine, and lumefantrine, offer alternative treatment options. Atovaquone-proguanil inhibits mitochondrial electron transport, while sulfadoxine-pyrimethamine interferes with folate synthesis. Lumefantrine exhibits similar action to chloroquine, though it maintains effectiveness in certain chloroquine-resistant strains. These drugs have their own unique profiles regarding efficacy, resistance, and side effects.

The development of resistance to antimalarials necessitates a multifaceted approach to disease management. This includes careful monitoring of parasite resistance patterns, rational drug use, and the development of new antimalarial compounds. Surveillance is essential for tracking changes in drug efficacy, and prompt adjustment of treatment guidelines is paramount to maintain control over malaria transmission. Regular updates and adaptation to regional changes are vital in effectively combating this disease.

Strategic deployment of antimalarial drugs, coupled with vector control measures, remains crucial in malaria control efforts. This involves responsible prescribing practices, strict adherence to treatment regimens, and public health initiatives aimed at improving sanitation, mosquito control, and early diagnosis. A comprehensive strategy, combining medication and preventative measures, represents the most effective approach to malaria control. Community involvement is crucial for effective implementation of these programs.

Beyond treatment, the importance of early diagnosis cannot be overstated. Rapid diagnostic tests (RDTs) and microscopy are invaluable tools for identifying malaria infections quickly and accurately. Prompt diagnosis and timely treatment significantly reduce the risk of severe complications and death. Early detection and treatment are critical for improving patient outcomes and reducing overall disease burden. RDTs are particularly useful in resource-limited settings due to their ease of use and portability.

The development of new antimalarial drugs and vaccines remains a high priority in global health research. Drug discovery efforts focus on identifying novel targets within the Plasmodium parasite, seeking to circumvent existing mechanisms of resistance. Vaccine development poses significant challenges, but recent advancements offer some promise. The ongoing research and development are essential in safeguarding future progress against this pervasive disease. The continuous quest for better treatments and prevention strategies is a testament to the commitment to eradicating malaria.

In conclusion, the fight against malaria requires a comprehensive, multi-pronged approach. This necessitates not only effective antimalarial drugs but also robust surveillance, responsible drug use, innovative research, and community-level engagement. Only through such coordinated efforts can we hope to make significant inroads against this persistent and deadly disease. This sustained effort promises a future where malaria is finally conquered.

5.2 Antiparasitic Agents

The effective treatment of parasitic infections relies heavily on a range of antiparasitic agents, each designed to target specific parasites or groups of parasites. These agents work through diverse mechanisms, exploiting vulnerabilities in the parasite's lifecycle or physiology. Understanding these mechanisms is crucial for effective treatment and minimizing the risk of drug resistance. For instance, some antiparasitic drugs interfere with the parasite's energy production, while others target its reproductive processes, preventing its multiplication and spread. The choice of drug depends heavily on the specific parasite involved, the location of the infection, and the patient's overall health, requiring careful diagnosis and consideration of potential side effects.

Many antiparasitic drugs, such as metronidazole, act by disrupting the parasite's DNA, thereby inhibiting its growth and reproduction. This direct action on the parasite's genetic material is particularly effective against certain protozoa and bacteria. Other drugs, like praziquantel, work by increasing the permeability of the parasite's cell membrane, causing it to lose vital ions and nutrients, ultimately leading to its death. This mechanism is effective against several types of helminths, particularly flatworms. The development of newer antiparasitic drugs often involves a complex process of drug discovery and development, guided by detailed knowledge of the parasite's biology. This includes identifying specific targets within the parasite, like enzymes or receptors, which can be disrupted by precisely designed compounds. The process is long and painstaking, often requiring extensive preclinical and clinical trials to ensure safety and effectiveness.

Furthermore, the administration of antiparasitic agents often requires precise dosage and timing to maximize efficacy while minimizing the risk of adverse effects. The duration of treatment can vary significantly depending on the type of parasite and its life cycle. For some infections, a single dose might suffice; others require multiple doses spread over several weeks or even months. Some antiparasitic drugs may be administered orally, while others may require injection or topical application. The choice of administration route will depend on several factors, including the type and severity of infection, the location of the infection, and the patient's overall health. A thorough understanding of pharmacokinetics and pharmacodynamics is crucial to optimize drug efficacy and minimize adverse effects.

Moreover, the development of drug resistance is a significant challenge in the treatment of parasitic infections. Parasites, like other microorganisms, can evolve mechanisms to overcome the effects of drugs. This can be through mutations that alter the drug target or through the development of efflux pumps that actively remove the drug from the parasite's cell. To combat this, researchers are constantly developing new drugs with novel mechanisms of action, and strategies for combining existing drugs are being explored. Combining drugs can make it more difficult for parasites to develop resistance, effectively acting as a preventative measure against the development of drug resistance. This approach can improve treatment outcomes and reduce the likelihood of recurrence.

In addition to traditional medications, alternative therapies are sometimes employed in conjunction with or as a complement to conventional antiparasitic treatments. These may include herbal remedies, nutritional supplements, or other complementary therapies. However, the efficacy of these alternative treatments is often not rigorously studied, and they should never replace conventional medical treatment without careful medical advice. It's important to remember that some herbal remedies may interact with conventional medications, potentially leading to adverse effects. Always consult a healthcare professional before using any alternative therapies in conjunction with conventional antiparasitic medications to ensure safe and effective treatment. A holistic approach, combining conventional medical treatment with lifestyle modifications and preventive measures, is usually more beneficial.

Finally, understanding the parasite's life cycle is critical for effective treatment. Many parasites have complex life cycles, involving multiple stages in different hosts. Targeting a particular stage in the lifecycle may prove particularly effective; for example, some drugs target the larval stages of a parasite, preventing its maturation and the development of clinical disease. Knowing the life cycle allows clinicians to implement control strategies to target the most vulnerable stage of the parasite, therefore increasing the chance of eliminating the parasite with a single course of treatment. Careful consideration of the parasite's life cycle, therefore, is vital for the optimal use of antiparasitic agents and the development of effective control strategies. The successful management of parasitic infections requires a multi-faceted approach, integrating advanced diagnostic techniques, a comprehensive understanding of the parasite's biology, and the judicious use of antiparasitic agents.

6 Evolutionary Arms Race

The constant interplay between parasite and host isn't a static conflict; it's a dynamic, ever-shifting arms race. This relentless evolutionary pressure has sculpted both parasite cunning and host resilience, a biological dance played out across millennia. Understanding this evolutionary tango is crucial to comprehending the complexities of parasitic diseases and devising effective strategies against them.

Consider the malaria parasite, Plasmodium falciparum. Its ability to rapidly switch its surface antigens, a classic example of antigenic variation, allows it to evade the host's adaptive immune response. Each time the immune system mounts a successful attack, the parasite has already shifted its identity, rendering the immune response largely ineffective. This continuous adaptation is a testament to the parasite's evolutionary prowess. The host, in turn, is driven to evolve a more sophisticated immune system capable of recognizing a wider range of parasite variants.

This co-evolutionary process isn't limited to antigenic variation.

Parasites often employ immune suppression techniques, actively dampening the host's immune response, creating an environment conducive to their survival and proliferation. They might secrete molecules that interfere with immune cell signaling pathways or directly inhibit immune cell function, effectively creating a haven within the host's body. This strategy, again, drives the evolution of more robust immune systems in the host population. The selective pressure exerted by the parasite leads to those hosts with more effective immune responses being more likely to survive and reproduce, passing these beneficial genes onto their offspring.

The implications of this evolutionary arms race extend far beyond the individual level. It shapes the population dynamics of both parasites and their hosts. Highly virulent parasites, while initially successful at rapid reproduction, may inadvertently harm their hosts so severely that transmission opportunities are reduced. This negative selection pressure favors parasites with less severe virulence, at least until other factors disrupt the balance. Consequently, the parasite's evolution becomes a delicate balance between exploitation and co-existence. A too-aggressive strategy can lead to the host's demise, taking the parasite with it.

Conversely, host populations with less effective immune systems face higher mortality rates from parasitic infections. This selection pressure, in turn, favors hosts with improved immune defenses. Thus, the evolutionary trajectory of both parasite and host is intrinsically linked, a dance of adaptation and counter-adaptation. This complex interaction means that any single point in time presents merely a snapshot of a much larger ongoing process.

Understanding the evolutionary history of host-parasite interactions is therefore critical for developing effective treatment strategies. Many antimalarial drugs, for instance, target specific metabolic pathways in the parasite, pathways that evolved long ago to fulfill a crucial role in the parasite's lifecycle. However, the very nature of the evolutionary arms race makes it difficult to win definitively. As new treatments emerge, parasites frequently adapt, developing resistance mechanisms, which in turn necessitates ongoing development of new drugs and therapeutic strategies. This illustrates how our medical interventions are often merely temporary shifts in a continuous evolutionary battle. The development of drug resistance highlights the profound necessity for understanding this ongoing evolutionary process. The understanding of parasite evolution allows for a more proactive approach to the development of new treatments and strategies.

The sophistication of parasite adaptations frequently surpasses our initial expectations. The capacity for adaptation in parasites demonstrates their remarkable ability to overcome environmental pressures. These pressures include not only the host's immune system, but also environmental conditions, such as climate change or changes in available food sources. Their adaptations frequently involve complex gene regulation, allowing for flexible responses to a vast array of conditions. Such adaptability further underscores the need for a long-term and multifaceted strategy in combating parasitic diseases, one that accounts for this constant evolutionary pressure.

Ultimately, understanding the evolutionary arms race between parasites and their human hosts reveals a fundamental truth: parasitic diseases are not static entities; they are dynamic systems shaped by millions of years of evolutionary pressure. This understanding forms the cornerstone of our efforts to develop effective treatments, vaccines and preventive strategies. Ignoring the evolutionary dimensions of these diseases would be akin to playing chess against an opponent who constantly changes the rules of the game - a battle that is practically unwinnable. The more deeply we understand the evolutionary intricacies of this host-parasite dance, the better equipped we will be to develop successful and long-lasting solutions.

6.1 Host-Parasite Coevolution

The intricate dance between host and parasite, a relentless evolutionary arms race, shapes the very nature of parasitic disease. This coevolutionary struggle isn't simply a static conflict; it's a dynamic process, constantly reshaping both parasite virulence and host resistance. Consider the malaria parasite, Plasmodium falciparum, its ability to switch surface antigens, a testament to its capacity to outmaneuver the host's adaptive immune system. This constant adaptation ensures the parasite's survival and propagation, perpetuating the cycle of infection and disease. Conversely, the human host, under selective pressure exerted by the parasite, develops a diverse array of immune defenses, striving to contain and eliminate the infection. This interplay between genetic variation in both host and parasite populations, coupled with environmental factors, influences the trajectory of disease transmission and severity. The outcome isn't predetermined; it's a consequence of this ongoing evolutionary pressure.

Understanding this coevolutionary dynamic is crucial for effectively combating parasitic diseases. A static approach to treatment, relying solely on existing drugs and therapies, risks becoming obsolete as parasites evolve resistance mechanisms. We must anticipate the parasite's evolutionary trajectory and develop proactive strategies. This requires a comprehensive understanding of parasite genetics, population dynamics, and the intricacies of host-parasite interactions at the molecular level. Research into the genetic basis of host resistance, for example, could pave the way for identifying individuals with naturally stronger defenses, providing insights into potential therapeutic targets.

Moreover, the geographic distribution of parasitic diseases is intimately linked to this ongoing coevolutionary process. Areas with high parasite prevalence frequently exhibit a higher frequency of host genes associated with resistance. Conversely, regions with low prevalence may display reduced resistance due to less selective pressure. This geographic variation highlights the importance of considering both ecological factors and the evolutionary history of host-parasite interactions when designing public health interventions. Understanding the selective pressures operating in different environments allows for more tailored and effective strategies in preventing and controlling the spread of parasitic diseases. A one-size-fits-all approach is unlikely to succeed in the face of such complexity.

The study of coevolution also provides invaluable insights into the evolution of virulence. While it might seem counterintuitive, parasites don't always benefit from maximal virulence. Excessively virulent parasites risk killing their hosts before they can effectively transmit to new hosts. This presents a trade-off: a balance between parasite replication and host survival. This balance is constantly being renegotiated, influenced by factors such as parasite transmission routes, population density, and the effectiveness of host immune responses. This understanding underpins the development of effective control measures. By modulating parasite transmission, for example through vector control or improved sanitation, we can potentially influence the selective pressures favoring less virulent strains.

Ultimately, mastering the complexities of host-parasite coevolution is paramount in the development of effective and sustainable disease control strategies. A deeper understanding of the evolutionary arms race isn't merely an academic pursuit; it forms the foundation of improved diagnostic tools, more effective drugs, and innovative prevention methods. The key lies in a holistic approach, integrating epidemiological surveillance, genetic analysis, and experimental studies of host-parasite interactions. By embracing the dynamic nature of this evolutionary struggle, we can hope to shift the balance in favor of the host and minimize the devastating impact of parasitic diseases on human health. This necessitates a dynamic, adaptable, and forward-thinking approach to combating parasitic diseases, forever recognizing the evolutionary pressures that shape this ongoing conflict. Therefore, research directed at understanding the evolutionary dynamics of host-parasite relationships is not simply a valuable endeavor; it's crucial for future success.

The ongoing arms race is an ever-changing landscape. The future of combating parasitic diseases demands a constant evaluation and adaptation of our strategies. We must proactively anticipate the emergence of resistant strains, and develop innovative approaches to treatment and prevention. Furthermore, advancements in genomic sequencing and bioinformatics are revolutionizing our ability to analyze parasite populations and monitor the evolution of resistance. This, coupled with improved epidemiological modeling, permits a more accurate prediction of disease outbreaks and more targeted interventions. The evolution of resistance to existing drugs is a sobering reminder that we cannot rest on our laurels in the field of parasitology. Continuous monitoring and development are paramount.

The development of new drugs and therapies is a critical aspect of this ongoing battle. Traditional approaches to drug discovery often focus on identifying compounds that target specific parasite pathways. However, the capacity of parasites to develop resistance to these targeted compounds necessitates a shift towards more innovative strategies. This involves exploring novel drug targets that are less prone to resistance development, as well as developing combination therapies to mitigate the effects of resistance. Furthermore, the understanding of host-parasite coevolution informs the development of new diagnostic tools, allowing for earlier detection and more effective treatment. These advancements are not merely incremental improvements; they are fundamental shifts in our ability to manage parasitic diseases effectively.

6.2 Adaptive Immunity

Adaptive immunity, the sophisticated, highly specific defense system, plays a crucial role in the intricate dance between parasite and host. Unlike the innate immune response's immediate, general reaction, adaptive immunity develops slowly, exhibiting specificity and immunological memory. This tailored response allows the body to learn and remember specific threats, mounting a stronger defense upon subsequent encounters. The key players here are lymphocytes, specifically B cells and T cells, both originating from hematopoietic stem cells in the bone marrow.

B cells, maturing primarily in the bone marrow, are responsible for antibody production. These antibodies, highly specific proteins, bind to parasite antigens—unique molecular structures on the parasite's surface. This binding neutralizes the parasite, marking it for destruction by other immune cells or complement proteins. The remarkable specificity arises from the extensive rearrangement of immunoglobulin genes during B cell development, creating a vast repertoire of potential antibodies. This ensures the immune system can adapt and recognize a nearly infinite number of potential parasitic threats. The process of affinity maturation, through somatic hypermutation and clonal selection, further refines the antibody's binding capacity throughout the immune response.

T cells, however, take a different but equally essential path. They mature in the thymus, undergoing rigorous selection processes to ensure self-tolerance and avoid attacking the host's own cells. Helper T cells (CD4+) coordinate the immune response, releasing cytokines that activate other immune cells, including B cells and cytotoxic T cells. Cytotoxic T cells (CD8+), on the other hand, directly kill infected cells, recognizing parasitic antigens presented on the surface of infected cells via major histocompatibility complex (MHC) class I molecules. This direct cellular destruction is pivotal in eradicating parasites that reside within host cells. Their actions are crucial in controlling parasitic infections that manage to bypass antibody-mediated defenses.

However, parasites, masters of evasion, have evolved ingenious mechanisms to subvert this powerful adaptive immune system. Antigenic variation, a common strategy, involves regularly altering surface antigens, effectively rendering antibodies useless against the shifted proteins. Immune suppression, another tactic, involves manipulating the host's immune response, actively downregulating cytokine production or directly targeting immune cells, thereby creating a window of opportunity for parasitic survival and proliferation. These parasitic strategies highlight the evolutionary arms race between pathogen and host, a relentless cycle of adaptation and counter-adaptation that shapes both immune and parasitic evolution.

Understanding this dynamic interaction is critical to developing effective therapies. Vaccines, for instance, exploit the principles of adaptive immunity, aiming to induce a protective immune response without causing disease. They typically introduce weakened or inactivated parasites, or parts thereof, to stimulate the production of specific antibodies and memory T cells, priming the body for future encounters with the parasite. However, successful vaccine development against many parasitic infections remains challenging due to their complex life cycles, antigenic variability, and the inherent challenges of creating effective immunogens. The development of novel drugs that either directly target parasite components or bolster the host's immune response is another active area of research, one that seeks to outmaneuver the ever-evolving strategies of parasitic organisms.

Furthermore, the intricacies of adaptive immunity in the context of parasitic infections are not fully understood. The role of regulatory T cells, for instance, in maintaining immune homeostasis and preventing excessive inflammation, requires further investigation. Similarly, the interplay between the innate and adaptive immune responses, and the precise mechanisms by which parasites evade each, deserve considerable attention. Understanding these aspects holds the key to developing more effective diagnostic tools and tailored treatment strategies. Ultimately, the better we understand the adaptive immune response and its manipulation by parasites, the more effectively we can combat these tenacious pathogens. The future of parasitic disease control lies in harnessing and augmenting the power of our adaptive immune system, a complex and crucial component in the unending battle between parasite and host.

6.3 Parasite Adaptation

The constant pressure exerted by the host's immune system drives parasites to evolve intricate adaptations, ensuring their survival and propagation. This evolutionary arms race is a dynamic process, shaped by natural selection favoring those parasites that can most effectively evade detection and manipulate their hosts. Consider the malaria parasite, Plasmodium falciparum, its ability to switch surface antigens, confusing the immune system and enabling repeated infections, is a testament to this relentless adaptation. This constant change makes developing effective vaccines incredibly challenging.

Many parasites have evolved mechanisms to directly suppress the host's immune response. For example, some helminths secrete molecules that actively dampen the inflammatory response, creating a more hospitable environment for their survival. This immune modulation is not simply a passive avoidance; it's an active manipulation of the host's biology, highlighting the sophistication of parasitic strategies. The immune system, while powerful, is not always successful in eliminating these invaders. Understanding these mechanisms is crucial for developing more effective treatments.

The environment also plays a significant role in parasite adaptation. Environmental changes, such as alterations in temperature, humidity, or resource availability, can selectively favor parasites with specific traits. For instance, climate change is predicted to impact the distribution and prevalence of various parasitic diseases, influencing which adaptations become advantageous. This underlines the complexity of parasitic evolution and its dependence on external factors. Predicting the future trajectory of parasitic diseases necessitates considering these environmental influences.

Some parasites have evolved remarkable mechanisms to manipulate host behavior, increasing their chances of transmission. For example, certain species of toxoplasmosis can alter the behavior of their rodent hosts, making them less cautious and more likely to be preyed upon by cats, the parasite's definitive host. This manipulation extends to other parasites, demonstrating the diversity of adaptations geared toward successful transmission. Such behavioral modifications are not random; they are the result of meticulous evolutionary refinement.

The ability to switch between different life cycle stages within the host or in the environment is another crucial adaptation for many parasites. This plasticity allows parasites to survive variations in host immunity, environmental conditions, or the availability of intermediate hosts. Such flexibility underscores the evolutionary resilience of parasitic organisms, ensuring their persistence in diverse and fluctuating environments. These intricate life cycle strategies are critical for their continued success.

Parasite adaptations are not limited to immune evasion or behavioral manipulation. Some parasites have evolved mechanisms to modify host cell structure, creating niches that enhance their own survival. They may alter cellular signaling pathways or gene expression profiles, creating a microenvironment conducive to their growth and reproduction. These cellular-level manipulations highlight the profound influence parasites can exert on their host's biology. Investigating these intricate processes can lead to novel therapeutic strategies.

Moreover, the development of drug resistance is a significant evolutionary challenge. The widespread use of antiparasitic drugs has inadvertently selected for drug-resistant strains, necessitating the constant development of new therapeutic agents. This ongoing "arms race" between humans and parasites necessitates continuous research and development efforts. The implications of this are substantial, as drug resistance compromises our ability to effectively manage and control parasitic infections.

Understanding parasite adaptation is paramount to developing effective strategies for disease prevention and treatment. Research focusing on the genetic basis of these adaptations, including genomic sequencing and comparative genomics, is helping us unravel the complex mechanisms underlying parasite evolution. This increased understanding will undoubtedly pave the way for innovative and more effective interventions. The continued investigation into these adaptations is vital.

7 Future Directions

The development of novel therapies represents a crucial frontier in combating parasitic diseases. Current treatments often suffer from limitations, including toxicity, drug resistance, and limited efficacy against certain parasites. Research into novel drug targets, such as parasite-specific enzymes or metabolic pathways, is essential. This includes exploring the potential of repurposing existing drugs for antiparasitic activity, leveraging computational modeling and high-throughput screening to identify novel compounds. Furthermore, investigating natural products and traditional medicine for antiparasitic compounds holds significant promise. The synergistic effect of combining different drugs to overcome resistance and improve treatment outcomes is also a focus of ongoing research. Success in this area necessitates a multidisciplinary approach, integrating expertise in chemistry, biology, pharmacology, and computational sciences. Understanding the specific mechanisms of action and resistance profiles of these novel therapies will be critical for their effective implementation.

Vaccine development against parasitic infections remains a significant challenge, particularly due to the complex life cycles and immune evasion strategies employed by many parasites. However, recent advancements in vaccine technology, including subunit vaccines, DNA vaccines, and attenuated parasites, offer renewed hope. The identification of protective antigens, those parts of the parasite that effectively elicit an immune response, is a major focus. Advancements in understanding the parasite's immunology and the host's immune response are equally crucial. It requires a clear delineation of the mechanisms through which effective immunity is achieved and sustained. Furthermore, addressing the challenges of vaccine delivery, particularly in resource-limited settings, is vital for ensuring widespread access to effective vaccines. Developing vaccines that target multiple stages of the parasite's life cycle could potentially provide more comprehensive protection, reducing the complexity of delivering multiple doses.

Research advancements are propelling the field forward, improving our understanding of parasite biology, host-parasite interactions, and disease pathogenesis. Advanced imaging techniques, such as confocal microscopy and electron microscopy, are providing increasingly detailed insights into the cellular mechanisms of parasite invasion and immune evasion. 'Omics' technologies, including genomics, transcriptomics, and proteomics, are enabling comprehensive analysis of parasite and host gene expression, allowing for the identification of novel drug targets and biomarkers. The use of advanced bioinformatics tools is paramount in interpreting this vast amount of data efficiently. Moreover, improved diagnostic tools are essential for early detection and effective management of parasitic infections. These improvements will lead to more targeted treatment strategies and better disease control. Studying the role of genetics, both parasite and host, in determining susceptibility to parasitic infections is a developing field; this data will also aid the creation of personalized treatment plans.

The integration of these three areas—novel therapies, vaccine development, and research advancements—is vital. The development of effective vaccines will reduce reliance on chemical therapies, minimizing the risk of drug resistance and toxicity. Improved diagnostic tools will enable more accurate assessments of infection severity and disease progression, leading to better treatment and vaccine effectiveness. Collaborative efforts between researchers, clinicians, and public health organizations are essential to translate these advancements into effective interventions and public health strategies. Ultimately, the future of combating parasitic diseases relies on sustained investment in research and development, coupled with international cooperation to overcome the challenges posed by these infections. Only then can we hope to significantly reduce the global burden of these debilitating and often fatal illnesses. This collaborative approach will allow us to create better diagnostics, treat those infected effectively, and ultimately prevent new infections.

7.1 Novel Therapies

The development of novel therapies for parasitic infections represents a crucial frontier in medical parasitology. Current treatments often suffer from limitations, including toxicity, drug resistance, and limited efficacy against certain parasite species. Therefore, exploring innovative therapeutic approaches is paramount. One promising area is the development of drugs targeting parasite-specific metabolic pathways. Many parasites rely on unique metabolic processes absent in humans, presenting opportunities for highly selective therapies with minimal side effects. For example, research into the unique folate metabolism of certain protozoa has yielded effective antifolate drugs. Similarly, targeting parasite-specific enzymes or proteins involved in essential processes like energy production or protein synthesis could lead to the creation of novel therapeutic agents.

Another avenue of research involves harnessing the power of the host immune system. Immunotherapies, which aim to boost or modulate the host's immune response against the parasite, are showing increasing promise. This could involve the use of monoclonal antibodies to target specific parasite antigens or the development of vaccines that stimulate a protective immune response. Harnessing the innate immune system, particularly through the activation of phagocytic cells like macrophages, may also provide a powerful strategy against intracellular parasites. The challenge lies in designing immunotherapies that are effective, safe, and adaptable to the diverse range of parasitic infections.

Gene editing technologies, like CRISPR-Cas9, offer revolutionary potential in combating parasitic diseases. These technologies could be used to modify the parasite's genome, making it less virulent or more susceptible to existing drugs. For example, disrupting genes essential for parasite survival or virulence could render them harmless or easily eliminated by the immune system. Conversely, gene editing could be employed to enhance the host's immune response by modifying genes involved in immune recognition or effector functions. However, ethical considerations surrounding gene editing in parasites and humans must be carefully addressed.

Furthermore, the use of nanotechnology in drug delivery holds considerable potential. Nanoparticles can be engineered to encapsulate antiparasitic drugs, targeting their delivery to specific sites within the host, improving drug efficacy and reducing side effects. This targeted delivery could also help overcome the problem of drug resistance, as higher concentrations of the drug can be achieved at the site of infection without systemic exposure. The development of smart nanoparticles that release their payload only upon reaching the target site further enhances the potential of this approach.

Naturally derived compounds, such as those found in plants and other organisms, represent a vast and largely untapped resource for discovering novel antiparasitic agents. Traditional medicine often uses plant-derived remedies against various parasitic infections, providing a rich foundation for identifying and characterizing bioactive compounds with antiparasitic activity. Screening natural product libraries for compounds with potent and selective antiparasitic effects could lead to the identification of new drug candidates. Importantly, this approach needs to be carefully integrated with modern drug development procedures to ensure safety and efficacy.

Finally, a multipronged approach is vital for achieving significant progress in the development of novel therapies. This includes a concerted effort to enhance our understanding of parasitic biology and pathogenesis, to conduct rigorous preclinical and clinical trials, and to foster collaborations between researchers in diverse fields, including parasitology, immunology, chemistry, and engineering. By combining traditional approaches with innovative technologies and methodologies, we can pave the way for more effective and safer treatments for parasitic infections, greatly improving global health outcomes. The future of combating parasitic diseases relies on creative and collaborative research, pushing the boundaries of medical science to create life-changing therapeutic options. Ultimately, a collaborative, multidisciplinary approach is needed. This involves not just drug development, but also improvements in diagnostics, public health initiatives, and an increased understanding of the complex interplay between parasites, their vectors, and their human hosts. Only through a comprehensive strategy can we hope to significantly reduce the global burden of parasitic diseases.

7.2 Vaccine Development

Developing effective vaccines against parasitic infections presents a significant challenge, unlike many viral or bacterial diseases. The complexity of parasite life cycles, their ability to manipulate host immune responses, and the diversity of parasitic species all contribute to this difficulty. However, advancements in our understanding of parasite immunology and vaccine technology offer promising avenues for future progress. One key strategy involves identifying parasite antigens capable of eliciting a strong and protective immune response. This requires extensive research, often involving sophisticated techniques like genomics and proteomics, to pinpoint specific molecules on the parasite's surface or within its cells that are highly immunogenic. These antigens must not only be highly conserved across different parasite strains but also capable of stimulating both humoral and cellular immunity for long-term protection.

A major hurdle is the parasitic ability to evade the immune system. Many parasites undergo antigenic variation, constantly changing their surface proteins to avoid recognition by antibodies. Others suppress the host's immune response, making it difficult for the vaccine to generate a protective effect. Therefore, vaccine design must consider these evasion strategies. Developing vaccines capable of generating broad and long-lasting immunity against these diverse and evasive pathogens requires a multi-pronged approach. This approach often focuses on targeting multiple parasite antigens simultaneously, or creating vaccines that stimulate different components of the immune system.

Subunit vaccines, using purified parasite proteins, offer a safer approach compared to whole-parasite vaccines. They eliminate the risk of infection from attenuated or inactivated parasites, a crucial advantage. However, subunit vaccines often require adjuvants to enhance their immunogenicity and stimulate a more robust immune response. The choice of adjuvant is vital, as it can significantly impact the effectiveness of the vaccine. This requires careful consideration of factors such as safety, immunogenicity, and compatibility with the chosen antigens. DNA vaccines hold promise for inducing both humoral and cellular immune responses, offering an alternative approach to traditional subunit vaccines. These vaccines deliver genetic material encoding parasite antigens directly into host cells, causing them to produce the antigens and stimulate an immune response.

Another challenge lies in the varying stages of parasite development. Many parasites have complex life cycles, involving different stages within the host and possibly in intermediate vectors. An effective vaccine needs to target the relevant stages that are crucial for transmission or pathogenesis. For instance, a vaccine targeting the sporozoite stage of malaria, the stage that infects humans, could be significantly more effective than one targeting the later blood stages. Furthermore, the efficacy of a vaccine can vary depending on the host's genetic background and pre-existing immunity. This necessitates population-specific vaccine design to ensure optimal effectiveness in different populations.

Furthermore, logistical challenges in vaccine delivery and implementation in endemic areas remain significant obstacles. Maintaining the cold chain for many vaccine types is often difficult in resource-limited settings. Therefore, developing vaccines that are thermostable, requiring minimal refrigeration, is essential for widespread implementation. The cost-effectiveness of vaccine production and distribution is also crucial. A vaccine must be affordable and accessible to the populations that need it most. Therefore, the development of vaccines against parasitic infections often involves a combination of advanced scientific research and careful consideration of public health factors. Ongoing research efforts focused on improving vaccine technology, alongside addressing these practical considerations, are essential to achieve meaningful progress in controlling these diseases. The complexities involved in vaccine development highlight the need for continued research and innovative strategies, moving towards a future where effective vaccines offer substantial protection against these pervasive and often devastating parasitic diseases.

7.3 Research Advancements

Next-generation sequencing technologies are revolutionizing our understanding of parasite genomes. High-throughput sequencing allows for the rapid and comprehensive identification of parasite genes, including those responsible for virulence, drug resistance, and immune evasion. This detailed genomic information is crucial for developing more effective diagnostic tools, targeted therapies, and preventative measures. Furthermore, comparative genomics across different parasite species reveals evolutionary relationships and conserved mechanisms that can be exploited in the development of broad-spectrum antiparasitic drugs. The ability to sequence entire parasite populations, rather than just single isolates, provides insights into genetic diversity and the potential for rapid adaptation, which is essential for anticipating and managing the emergence of drug resistance. This data-driven approach is transforming our ability to understand and combat parasitic infections.

Proteomics offers a powerful complementary approach to genomics, focusing on the parasite's protein profile. Mass spectrometry allows researchers to identify and quantify thousands of proteins expressed by a parasite at any given time. This reveals the complex interplay of proteins involved in parasite development, host-parasite interactions, and disease pathogenesis. Mapping these proteins to specific pathways provides valuable targets for drug development, as inhibiting key proteins can disrupt crucial parasite functions without harming the host. The integration of proteomics data with genomic information provides a holistic view of the parasite's biology and offers a more comprehensive understanding of its interaction with the human host. This integrated approach has proven particularly useful in identifying novel drug targets and biomarkers for early disease detection.

Advanced imaging techniques, such as confocal microscopy and electron microscopy, provide high-resolution visualization of parasite-host interactions at the cellular level. This allows researchers to observe parasite invasion mechanisms, immune responses, and the effects of parasitic infection on host cells in real-time. Three-dimensional imaging allows for detailed reconstruction of parasite structures and their interaction with host tissues, providing unprecedented insight into the dynamic processes involved in parasitic infections. Moreover, fluorescent labeling techniques enable the specific tracking of individual parasite proteins or host immune cells, providing valuable information about the precise interactions involved in disease progression. These detailed images often provide critical information that complement genomic and proteomic data, leading to a deeper understanding of disease mechanisms.

Bioinformatics plays an increasingly important role in analyzing the vast amounts of data generated by genomic, proteomic, and imaging studies. Sophisticated algorithms and machine learning techniques are used to identify patterns, predict protein functions, and model parasite-host interactions. These computational tools are essential for managing and interpreting large datasets, identifying potential drug targets, and predicting the evolution of parasite populations. The development of user-friendly bioinformatics tools is making these powerful techniques accessible to a broader range of researchers, facilitating collaborative research efforts and accelerating the pace of discovery. This computational approach is vital in connecting various research findings into a unified understanding of the complexity of parasitic infections.

The development of humanized mouse models and other in vivo systems allows researchers to study parasitic infections in a more realistic setting, mimicking the complexity of human immune responses and disease progression. These models provide an essential bridge between in vitro studies and clinical trials, validating promising therapeutic targets and facilitating the preclinical development of new drugs and vaccines. By manipulating genetic factors in these models, scientists can investigate the specific roles of individual genes in parasite virulence and host susceptibility, providing valuable insights into disease mechanisms and potential therapeutic approaches. Furthermore, the use of humanized models reduces the ethical concerns associated with using animal models that are less relevant to human biology, ensuring the relevance and reliability of research findings.

Finally, collaborative research efforts involving multiple disciplines, including parasitology, immunology, genomics, proteomics, and bioinformatics, are crucial for accelerating progress in the field. International collaborations are essential for sharing data, resources, and expertise, leading to a more comprehensive and efficient approach to combating parasitic diseases. Open access data sharing and the development of standardized research protocols further enhance the collaborative effort. This integrated approach leverages the strengths of each discipline, accelerating the discovery of novel diagnostic tools, therapeutics, and preventive strategies. Such collaborative advancements are fundamental to creating a more effective and global approach to the study and treatment of parasitic infections.

www.ingramcontent.com/pod-product-compliance
Lightning Source LLC
LaVergne TN
LVHW022015200926
848481LV00007B/2396